for beginners

AI in Healthcare for Beginners

Discover How Artificial Intelligence is Transforming Medical Diagnosis, Treatment, and Research

Printed in the United States of America

First Edition: 2025

This copyright page includes the necessary copyright notice, permissions request information, acknowledgments for the cover design, interior design, and editing, as well as the details of the first edition.

www.littlebiggiant.com

Introduction

The clinic room smelled like coffee and printer ink. A small machine hummed on the counter. It had just finished scanning a child's eye and spit out a paper with a word on it. The nurse read it out loud. The word was "refer." The child's mother went still. Her hand tightened on the paper. The doctor had not yet walked in. The machine had done what doctors sometimes missed. In 2018, the U.S. Food and Drug Administration authorized an AI system called IDx-DR to detect diabetic retinopathy from eye scans without a specialist looking first. It was the first time an AI device was cleared to give a medical result on its own. That one sentence changed more than the paper in the nurse's hand. It left the room quieter, heavier.

"What if the machine is wrong?" the mother asked, voice flat and small. The nurse looked at her. The kid blinked hard and swallowed. The doctor entered with a calm voice. The calm was not the same as the old kind of calm. This one carried tools no one could see. Machines now read pictures. Machines now spot patterns faster than the eye alone. That can mean a problem found early. It can also mean a new kind of worry. Machines learn from lots of data. They do not feel. They do not promise. They only give answers based on what they have been shown. AI in Healthcare for Beginners: Discover How Artificial Intelligence is Transforming

Medical Diagnosis, Treatment, and Research will take readers into moments like this. It will show how an answer from a machine can be a lifeline. It will show how it can be a question that keeps people awake at night. Hands hold papers. Eyes search faces. Voices ask simple, urgent things. Who decides when the machine's voice is the one to trust? Who catches what the machine misses? The paper waits on the counter and the room waits with it.

Table of Contents

Chapter 1

Foundations of AI in Healthcare

Outcome: By the end of this chapter you will be able to explain in simple terms how AI works in medicine, what kinds of models and data drive it, and how history shapes today's possibilities.

1. What artificial intelligence means for medicine: models, algorithms, and data

You will begin by seeing AI as three interlocking parts. The first part is models. Think of a model as a map that tries to predict or decide something, based on patterns it learned from many examples. A model could look at pictures of lungs to say whether a shadow is more likely to be a pneumonia or something else. The second part is algorithms. An algorithm is the set of rules that tells the model how to learn and how to make decisions when new information comes in. Some algorithms are simple and some are complex, but they all follow a plan or recipe to interpret data and produce results. The third part is data. Data is the raw material AI learns from: patient records, medical images, notes from doctors, lab results, and more. The quality, diversity, and size of this data shape how well the model can learn useful patterns.

A simple way to picture this is to imagine teaching a student to recognize a disease from photos. You would gather many labeled pictures, show them to the student, and point out which ones show the disease and which don't. The student learns a rule from those examples, and when a new photo comes along, the student uses the rule to guess whether the disease is present. In AI, the rules are learned automatically. The patient benefit is not from a single photo but from a long training process that uses thousands or millions of examples to find patterns that humans might miss.

Two brief micro-cases help this click into place. In one clinic, a machine-learning model looks at chest X-rays and flags possible pneumonia for a radiologist to review. The model doesn't replace the radiologist; it speeds up the process by focusing attention on the cases most likely to need a human check. In another setting, an AI tool combs through heart test results and historical outcomes to estimate a patient's risk of a future heart event, helping clinicians decide who might benefit most from preventive therapy. These examples show how models, when paired with good data and careful testing, can support real clinical decisions rather than replace doctors.

Yet you should notice three caveats that often appear with this first point. First, data quality matters a lot. If the data contain errors, gaps, or biases, the model can learn the wrong lessons. Second, models don't understand medicine the way humans do; they detect patterns but don't grasp meaning or context in the same way a clinician does. Third, models must be used with care: they provide information and probabilities, not guarantees. The goal is to combine the speed and scale of AI with human judgment, mercy, and clinical insight.

2. Brief history and major milestones in medical AI development

History in medicine moves from simple ideas to more powerful systems, but it always serves human judgment. In the earliest days, people built rule-based programs that mimicked expert thinking. One famous example was a system that assisted with infectious-disease decisions; it relied on a curated set of rules drawn from medical knowledge. These early efforts showed that computers could formalize professional reasoning and help with difficult choices, but they also revealed limits—rules could be brittle, and adapting them to new situations required human experts to rework the logic.

A second wave arrived when researchers started using statistical methods to learn from data. Instead of hand-crafting every rule, the computer learned patterns from many examples. This shift opened doors to recognizing complex signals in data, such as subtle patterns in images or patient histories that humans might miss.

The modern era of rapid progress began with deep learning, a kind of machine learning that learns from very large amounts of data and can handle complex, high-dimensional inputs like images and text. A landmark moment came when a breakthrough model made dramatic gains in image recognition, sparking widespread interest in applying similar ideas to medical images. Since then, many clinics and research centers have explored AI in radiology, pathology, and beyond, always starting from the question: will this help patients and fit into real-world care?

Two micro-cases illustrate how milestones translate to everyday practice. In the 1970s, a system named MYCIN explored how computers could help with infectious-disease decisions. It didn't become a routine clinical tool, but it showed that computers could encode medical knowledge to assist clinicians. In the 2010s, researchers moved from small datasets to larger collections of medical images and patient records, allowing deep-learning models to detect patterns with performance closer to or exceeding human benchmarks in certain tasks. These advances didn't erase the need for clinicians; they shifted the workload toward tasks where AI can provide speed, consistency, and scale.

Understanding this history helps you see why today's opportunities feel so compelling and why you should stay grounded. Technology moves quickly, but medicine is patient-facing and risk-averse. The best AI tools emerge when developers, clinicians, and patients share goals and work through validation, calibration, and governance together. This collaborative path keeps the momentum while preserving safety, trust, and accountability.

3. Realistic assessment of opportunities, limitations, and hype

Now you turn to what AI can realistically do in medicine and what it cannot do yet. The opportunities you should expect are substantial, but they come with clear boundaries.

What AI can do well

- Accelerate pattern recognition across large datasets. AI can sift through thousands of images, notes, or test results faster than a person and flag unusual or high-risk cases for review.

- Support decision-making with probabilities and explanations. Clinicians can use AI to see potential risks, compare treatment options, and check for consistency with patient data.

- Enhance consistency and workflow. AI can standardize measurements, automate repetitive tasks like data extraction, and help integrate information from different sources into one view for clinicians.

- Speed up research and discovery. By scanning many publications, datasets, and trial results, AI can help scientists identify promising hypotheses and accelerate biomarker discovery or drug repurposing.

What AI cannot do yet (and why)

- Understand context the way a human does. AI does not grasp the social, emotional, and ethical dimensions of care on its own, so human judgment remains essential.

- Generalize perfectly to new patients or settings. If data come from one hospital or one patient group, the AI's performance may drop in a different hospital with a different population or equipment.

- Replace safety, oversight, and regulation. Decisions about patient care still require clinical responsibility, clear consent, robust validation, and appropriate governance.

Where hype can mislead you

- People may promise dramatic breakthroughs overnight. Real progress often comes in incremental steps, with careful testing and integration into real-world workflows.

- There is a tendency to conflate correlation with causation. AI might find patterns that correlate with outcomes, but that doesn't always reveal why something happens or what to do about it.

- It's easy to overstate capabilities in unproven areas. For example, AI may excel at a narrow diagnostic task in a controlled study but struggle with the messy variability of everyday practice.

Two micro-cases of opportunity and limitation help you see the balance. In a busy clinic, an AI tool can help a physician triage patients by flagging those who most need urgent attention, speeding up care for everyone. But in the same setting, a model trained mainly on one population may misjudge risk for patients who look different in age, ethnicity, or medical history, leading to wrong priorities unless clinicians review and adjust it. In research, AI can rapidly scan thousands of papers to identify potential drug targets, yet translating those targets into safe, effective treatments still requires rigorous experiments, clinical trials, and regulatory oversight. These examples show the promise of AI, paired with careful testing, real-world validation, and ongoing collaboration.

An honest look at opportunity and risk helps you plan better. If you want AI to help in medicine, you should start with clear goals, collect diverse and high-quality data, and work in close partnership with clinicians and patients. Build validation into every step: test the model on new patients, monitor performance over time, and update it as care patterns change. Guard against bias by asking who is represented in the data and who might be left out. Always pair AI outputs with human interpretation rather than treating them as decisions in themselves. Finally, invest in governance: transparent development, documentation of how models are trained, and thoughtful policies about privacy, consent, and accountability.

Coming up next, you will dive into the specifics of Healthcare Data Types and Management. You'll explore how electronic records, imaging, wearables, registries, and genomic datasets shape what AI can learn, how data quality matters, and why privacy-preserving methods and governance frameworks matter for sensitive information. In this next chapter, you'll learn how data becomes the fuel for the smart tools you've just started to understand, and you'll see how to approach data with the same care you bring to patient care.

Key Takeaway: AI in medicine works by learning from lots of real data through models guided by algorithms, and its power grows when clinicians guide, validate, and govern its use.

Coming up next: Healthcare Data Types and Management—electronic health records, imaging, wearables, registries, and genomic datasets; data quality, annotation practices, and interoperability challenges; privacy-preserving methods and governance frameworks for sensitive data.

Chapter 2

Healthcare Data Types and Management

You will learn the main healthcare data types, why data quality matters, and how privacy protections keep patient information safe while AI can help doctors.

Electronic health records, imaging, wearables, registries, and genomic datasets

In hospitals and clinics, people collect data to tell the story of a patient's health. Electronic health records, or EHRs, are like digital notebooks that hold a patient's medical history: visits, diagnoses, medicines, lab results, allergies, and sometimes notes from doctors. EHRs help teams stay on the same page, even if a patient sees different doctors or changes clinics.

Imaging is another big source of data. X-rays, CT scans, MRIs, and ultrasound pictures capture what's happening inside the body. Each image is a picture with meaning that trained eyes can read, and increasingly, computer systems can help read those images too. Imaging data often comes with measurements, annotations, and reports that describe what the image shows.

Wearables are devices that people wear on their bodies—wristbands, chest patches, or smart watches—that collect information like heart rate, activity, sleep, and sometimes glucose or blood oxygen levels. Wearables give a daily stream of data, not just a snapshot from a clinic visit. They help show trends over weeks or months.

Registries collect data about groups of patients with the same condition or treatment. They track outcomes over time across many clinics. For example, a registry for a specific cancer might collect information about treatments, side effects, and survival, helping researchers see which approaches work best in the real world.

Genomic datasets hold DNA information. These datasets can reveal inherited risks, how a person might respond to certain drugs, or why a disease behaves differently in different people. Genomic data adds a deeper, biological layer to what clinicians observe in symptoms and tests.

Two micro-cases illustrate how these data types can work together. Micro-case one: a hospital team wants to flag patients who are at risk of kidney problems after a new medication. They pull EHR data to see age, existing conditions, medications, and lab results, and they bring in imaging notes when available to check for early signs of organ stress. The goal is to identify those patients early enough to adjust treatment or monitor them more closely. Micro-case two: a research group studies which patients with a particular autoimmune disease respond best to a new therapy. They combine data from disease registries, genomic datasets, and EHRs, then examine how genetic markers and previous treatments relate to outcomes. The combination helps researchers spot patterns that one data source alone might miss.

All these data types have a common purpose: to give a fuller, more accurate view of a person's health. When used well, they can reveal connections that aren't obvious from a single source. When used poorly, they can mislead, especially if information is missing, out of date, or recorded in incompatible ways. That's why data quality and how data fits together matter as much as the data itself.

Data quality, annotation practices, and interoperability challenges

Data quality is about how good the data is for your purpose. In health data, you care about accuracy (is the information correct?), completeness (is enough information there to tell the story?), timeliness (is it up to date?), and consistency (do similar entries look the same across systems and over time?). Real clinics see problems like missing values in a lab result, duplicate records for the same visit, or a medication list that doesn't match between an EHR and a pharmacy system. These problems aren't just annoying; they can lead to wrong conclusions or missed patient needs.

Annotation practices help machines understand data. Annotation means labeling data in a way that a computer can learn from. For imaging, annotation might mean drawing circles around a tumor and naming its type. For clinical notes, annotation could involve tagging symptoms, procedures, or tasks so a learning model can recognize patterns.

Good annotations require clear definitions, consistency across annotators, and careful review so the labels match what clinicians mean in real life.

Interoperability is the ability for different systems to share data smoothly. Many clinics use different software, and they might store the same information in different formats or under different codes. This makes it hard to combine data from one source with data from another. A common path forward is to adopt shared standards and careful mapping between systems. For example, imaging often uses standardized file formats, while patient data in EHRs benefits from standardized codes and fields that many systems recognize. When teams speak a common language, data can blend more reliably and be compared across places.

Two more micro-cases help bring this to life. Micro-case three: two hospitals try to combine patient records to study a rare side effect of a drug. One hospital uses one coding system for diagnoses, the other uses a different one. They invest time in mapping the codes and standardizing the data dictionary so the two datasets can talk to each other. The effort pays off when researchers can see a clearer signal across the larger group. Micro-case four: a national registry collects information from clinics that use different EHR vendors. To keep data useful, the team builds a shared data dictionary and trains staff on how to enter key fields in the same way every time, improving consistency across the entire registry.

If you want to improve data quality in a real project, a few practical steps help a lot. Step 1: Define clear data quality goals for your use case. Decide what matters most—accuracy, timeliness, or a particular completeness criterion—and keep that in focus. Step 2: Build automated checks that surface missing values, obvious errors, or inconsistencies. Regularly review flagged issues and correct the root causes, not just the symptoms. Step 3: Create a data dictionary that explains what every field means, what codes are used, and how to interpret each value. This dictionary acts as a guide for everyone who touches the data. Step 4: Develop a simple map or bridge between systems so data from one source can be translated into the standard format used in your project. When you have clear definitions and reliable mappings, data from many places can be combined with confidence.

A practical challenge to watch for is bias in data. If one clinic serves a particular community and records in a certain way, the data you collect from that clinic can color your results more than you expect. It's not a flaw in a single dataset; it's a signal to examine how representative your data truly is and whether you need additional sources to balance it. Being vigilant about representativeness helps keep AI tools fair and useful for everyone.

Privacy-preserving methods and governance frameworks for sensitive data

Safeguarding patient privacy is essential in every data project. Even with large, rich datasets, you need ways to protect people's identities and to control who can see or use the data. Broadly, privacy-preserving methods aim to reduce risk while preserving enough information to be useful. One basic approach is de-identification, which removes obvious identifiers like names and addresses. Yet de-identification is not a perfect shield—careful data handling, thoughtful data minimization, and thoughtful sharing agreements are still required because some information can still reveal someone's identity when combined with other data.

Good governance frameworks add structure and accountability. A governance framework outlines who owns the data, who can access it, for what purposes, and under what conditions. It often includes policies, consent considerations, and oversight steps. Common elements include data-use agreements that spell out allowed uses, data access controls so only authorized people can see sensitive information, and regular audits to verify that the rules are followed. Institutions may also involve review boards or ethics committees to consider patient protections and risk.

Two micro-cases illustrate privacy and governance in action. Micro-case five: a hospital team wants to use de-identified EHR data to train a machine learning model that predicts readmission risk. They remove direct identifiers, apply safeguards to reduce the chance of re-identification, and require researchers to sign a data-use agreement that limits how the data can be used and who can access it. Micro-case six: a research partnership wants to combine data from multiple clinics to study treatment outcomes while protecting patient privacy. They implement governance steps that document who can access the data, how data will be shared, and what safeguards are in place, including secure environments for analysis and clear data-retention rules.

If you're putting privacy into practice, here are some straightforward steps. Step 1: Map how data flows through your project—from collection to storage to analysis—so you know where sensitive information lives. Step 2: Define who can access the data and why. Use the principle of least privilege: give people the minimum access they need to do their work. Step 3: Talk with patients and families about how their data might be used. Collect consent where it makes sense and keep records of what was decided. Step 4: Put in place clear data-use agreements and governance processes that describe allowed purposes, data protection measures, and how problems will be handled. Step 5: Set up auditing and logging so you can track who accessed data and what they did with it. These steps don't just protect people; they also build trust with patients, clinicians, and researchers.

When data are high quality, well annotated, and governed by solid privacy rules, you unlock a lot of potential. You can combine information from many sources to spot patterns that help doctors diagnose earlier, tailor treatments, and learn what works best for different patients. But without these guardrails, you risk mistakes, privacy breaches, or lost trust, which can halt promising work before it begins.

Key Takeaway: Good data means good decisions—clear data types, clean quality, and strong privacy rules create a foundation where AI can help without risking people's safety or trust.

Coming up next: Core Machine Learning Concepts for Clinicians

1) Supervised, unsupervised, and reinforcement learning explained with examples

2) Training pipelines, validation strategies, and avoiding overfitting

3) Explainability methods and interpreting model outputs for clinical use

In the next chapter, you'll see how these ideas turn data into practical tools. You'll learn simple, concrete examples that show how doctors can use learning methods to read models, trust their outputs, and apply insights safely in real patient care. You'll also discover common traps and how to parse model results so they support good clinical decisions rather than confuse them.

Chapter 3

Core Machine Learning Concepts for Clinicians

By the end of this chapter, you will understand three core machine learning concepts clinicians actually use: supervised, unsupervised, and reinforcement learning; how to build training pipelines and validation to avoid overfitting; and how explainability helps you interpret model outputs in real clinical settings.

1. Understand the three learning types

Supervised learning means the model learns from examples that already have the right answer. Each input comes with a label, like a photo of a chest X-ray labeled "pneumonia" or "no pneumonia." The model tries to predict that label for new images and gets better as it sees more labeled pairs. In a hospital setting, supervised learning is often used to predict outcomes or classify findings from images or notes, because there is a clear answer to learn from.

Unsupervised learning looks for patterns in data without labels. The data have inputs but no correct outputs. The model tries to find structure—groups, clusters, or latent patterns—so you can spot new or hidden relationships. In medicine, unsupervised learning can reveal patient subgroups that share similar symptoms or lab profiles, which helps tailor care even when you don't know the exact labels ahead of time.

Reinforcement learning learns by trial and feedback. An agent takes actions in an environment and receives rewards or punishments that guide future choices. The goal is to maximize total reward over time. In healthcare, reinforcement learning is discussed as a way to improve decision sequences, such as planning treatment steps or dosing strategies, by learning from simulated trials and real-world feedback.

Step 1: Read the three types aloud until you can describe them in your own words. The goal is a mental map you can recall under pressure. Step 2: Match the task to the type. If you have clear labeled outcomes to predict, think supervised. If you want to discover patterns without labels, consider unsupervised. If the job is about choosing a sequence of actions and learning from the outcomes, reinforcement learning is the right frame. Step 3: Think of clinical flavor. Supervised learning is common in image and text classification; unsupervised helps with grouping and discovery; reinforcement learning sits at the edge of optimizing long-term strategies. Step 4: Note the limits. Supervised models depend on quality and breadth of labels; unsupervised models depend on meaningful patterns rather than predefined answers; reinforcement learning requires careful setup to avoid unsafe or unrealistic trial feedback.

Micro-case A (supervised): You have a dataset of chest X-rays labeled as "pneumonia" or "no pneumonia." You train a model to recognize signs of infection in the images and then test it on new X-rays. The aim is faster triage in busy clinics, supporting clinicians with a second opinion. The model's predictions come with confidence scores so you can decide when to trust its judgment and when to review manually. In this setup, success means accurate labeling on new images and useful help for decision-making, not full replacement of human judgment.

Micro-case B (unsupervised): You collect notes and lab results from thousands of patients but without labeled outcomes. You run an unsupervised clustering algorithm and find several patient groups that share similar symptoms and lab patterns. These clusters don't tell you which group is "better" or "worse," but they reveal distinct profiles that might respond differently to treatment. The insight can guide research ideas and personalized care plans without needing a labeled target from the start.

2. Build training pipelines and validate to prevent overfitting

Step 5: Outline a simple pipeline. Gather data, clean it, and decide what you want the model to do.

Split the data into a training portion to teach the model and a validation portion to check its progress. If you need a final check, reserve a test set to see how the model does on entirely new data. Keep track of how the data are prepared, since small changes can change outcomes a lot.

Step 6: Pick a validation strategy. A straightforward hold-out split gives you a rough read on performance. If you have more data, cross-validation averages performance over several splits for a more stable estimate. In healthcare, you also want to test on data from a different hospital or a different time period to see if the model generalizes beyond one dataset. External validation is especially important when patient populations or imaging devices vary.

Step 7: Avoid overfitting. Overfitting happens when a model learns the training data too well and fails on new data. Use simpler models when possible, and favor features that matter clinically rather than every possible detail. Techniques like regularization add a gentle penalty for complexity. Early stopping halts training when performance on validation data stops improving. Data augmentation—slightly changing images or text to create more examples—can help models learn to generalize. Always monitor both training and validation performance; if the gap grows, you likely need to adjust.

Step 8: Practical notes and caveats. Real clinical data are messy: missing values, mislabeled cases, and biased samples can mislead a model. Document how you handle missing data and why. When you report performance, include not just accuracy but also other measures that matter for healthcare, such as sensitivity (catching true positives) and specificity (not mislabeling healthy cases). Remember that a model's usefulness is as much about how it fits into workflow as about numbers on a scorecard.

3. Explainability: interpreting model outputs for clinical use

Step 9: Distinguish between explainable and interpretable models. Some models are inherently easy to understand, like simple decision trees. Others are more complex, like deep neural networks, and require post-hoc explanations to show what influenced a prediction. Both paths matter in medicine, where you need to understand why a decision was made.

Explainability tools come in two broad families. Interpretable models print a straightforward path to a result. Post-hoc explanations, used after the fact, highlight which features most influenced a decision. Methods such as SHAP values or partial dependence plots help you see how different inputs push the output in a certain direction. Use these tools to check whether the model's reasoning makes sense in clinical terms.

Step 10: Read outputs with care. A model might assign a high risk score to a patient who looks healthy, or miss a subtle sign in a rare case. Treat explanations as guides, not guarantees. Use them to identify where the model agrees with you and where it disagrees. Always verify with your clinical judgment and available patient history. Calibrate predictions with real-world outcomes, and be ready to adjust thresholds to match the level of risk your setting is comfortable managing.

Step 11: Communicate and manage expectations. Explainability helps you discuss model results with colleagues and patients. Present the main drivers behind a prediction in plain language, and describe what you will do next—whether it's collecting more data, ordering an additional test, or adjusting a treatment plan. Be transparent about uncertainties and the limits of the model. Remember, the goal is to support, not replace, human expertise.

Troubleshooting note: common pitfalls include relying on a single metric, ignoring generalizability, and misinterpreting explanations as proofs. Quick fixes include reporting multiple metrics, validating on diverse data, and using explainability results as a check on the model's logic rather than a final verdict.

Key Takeaway: You gain a practical map for three core machine learning concepts, learn how to build safe, generalizable training pipelines, and develop a disciplined approach to reading and using model explanations in patient care.

Coming up next: AI in Medical Imaging and Pathology

1) Automated image analysis for radiology, histopathology, and ophthalmology

2) Clinical validation studies, performance metrics, and comparative benchmarking

3) Deployment considerations for picture archiving systems and imaging workflows

Chapter 4

AI in Medical Imaging and Pathology

By the end of this chapter, you will understand how AI helps analyze medical images in three key areas: automated image analysis across radiology, histopathology, and ophthalmology; how researchers test these tools with validation studies and performance metrics; and what clinics consider when deploying imaging AI within picture archiving and workflow systems.

Automated image analysis for radiology, histopathology, and ophthalmology

Step 1: Define what you are trying to find in the image. In radiology, AI looks for shapes or patterns that may indicate disease, such as a suspicious shadow in a chest X-ray or an abnormal growth on a CT scan. In histopathology, AI scans slides of tissue to help identify cancer cells, tissue structure, or unusual patterns. In ophthalmology, AI examines eye photos to spot signs of vision-threatening conditions like diabetic retinopathy. The common thread is that the tool learns to distinguish typical patterns from unusual ones, so clinicians can focus on the cases that matter most. The goal is not to replace a clinician's eye, but to extend it with careful, repeatable analysis.

Step 2: Learn how the outputs look and what they mean. When you use automated image analysis, outputs often include highlighted regions, probability scores, or label suggestions. The highlighted areas point to where the model thinks something noteworthy might be. The probability score gives a sense of confidence—how sure the tool is about its guess. A label might say "suspicious nodule" or "cancer-positive region." You interpret these results as guidance, not final judgment. Always cross-check with your own experience and the patient's overall picture. This collaboration between human and machine is where AI shines.

Step 3: See how the tools fit into real clinical tasks. In radiology, an AI aid might flag potential nodules on a chest X-ray so you can review them more quickly. In histopathology, it can triage slides so a pathologist sees the most urgent cases first. In ophthalmology, it can screen large populations and identify patients who need a closer look. The simplest rule is to start with tasks that have clear, measurable benefits: faster triage, reduced missed findings, or standardized lay-in readings. The strongest tools hand back control to clinicians, keeping the human in the loop for interpretation and decision-making.

Examples and micro-cases

Micro-case 1: A radiology clinic uses an AI tool to help flag small nodules on chest X-rays. The system marks several regions and assigns confidence scores. A radiologist reviews the flagged images, confirming two true positives and dismissing one false alarm. The tool reduces the time spent scanning every image, especially on busy days, while maintaining high accuracy.

Micro-case 2: A pathology lab trains an AI model to sort tissue slides by likely cancer presence. One batch of slides shows clear patterns that align with what a pathologist already looks for, while another batch reveals new cellular textures the human eye initially misses. The pathologist uses the AI as a first read to prioritize urgent cases and then applies standard checks to confirm results.

Micro-case 3: In an eye clinic, fundus photographs are analyzed to detect signs of diabetic retinopathy. The AI highlights areas of abnormal vessels and bleeding, and clinicians review the highlighted patterns alongside patient history. This approach helps catch issues early in patients who may not notice subtle vision changes, enabling earlier care.

Clinical validation studies, performance metrics, and comparative benchmarking

Step 1: Understand what validation means for imaging AI. Validation studies test how well a tool works on data that wasn't used to train it. They often use separate sets of images from different sources to show that the tool can generalize beyond its original training. The most trustworthy validations show results on data that resemble real patient cases and reflect typical clinical workflows. The aim is to demonstrate usefulness in practice, not just in a lab.

Step 2: Learn the common metrics and what they tell you. You will hear terms like sensitivity (how often the tool catches a real positive), specificity (how often it correctly ignores a real negative), and AUC or area under the curve (overall ability to separate positives from negatives). There may also be accuracy, precision, and recall, or calibration measures that show whether the tool's probability scores line up with real outcomes. Different tasks emphasize different metrics. For screening, sensitivity is often prioritized; for confirming a diagnosis, specificity can be key. Remember that a single number rarely tells the full story—look at patterns across several metrics and in diverse data.

Step 3: Compare AI to humans and to older tools. Comparative benchmarking asks: does the AI tool perform as well as a clinician, or better in specific tasks? How does it compare to existing software? Does it hold up on new image types or images from different hospitals? Benchmarking helps you see strengths and limits. It also guides where the AI should act as a helper rather than a replacement. A fair comparison uses the same task definitions, the same kinds of images, and a clear description of what success looks like.

Examples and micro-cases

Micro-case 1: A study compares an AI chest X-ray tool with radiologists on detecting a common lung finding. The AI identifies many true positives and some misses, while radiologists catch other cases that AI misses. The combined approach improves overall detection, showing the value of AI as a second reader rather than a replacement.

Micro-case 2: An AI system for retinal images is benchmarked against ophthalmologists for grading disease severity. The tool's performance aligns with human experts on several categories and explains its predictions with simple visual maps. Clinicians use this information to triage patients and plan follow-up visits more efficiently.

Micro-case 3: A pathology workflow tests an AI slide classifier on multiple labs. Results show consistent performance across centers, but some slide preparation differences lead to performance shifts. The team includes calibration steps to adjust the tool for each lab's data, maintaining reliability across sites.

Deployment considerations for picture archiving systems and imaging workflows

Step 1: Know what PACS and imaging workflows are. Picture Archiving and Communication Systems (PACS) store, retrieve, and display medical images. An AI tool in this setting should integrate with the same workflow, so results appear in the clinician's usual view alongside the images. The goal is a smooth experience where AI findings feel like an extra set of eyes rather than an extra manual step.

Step 2: Plan for integration, safety, and privacy. Ensure the AI tool speaks the same language as your imaging system, using standard formats and safe data handling. Consider who can access results, how patient information is protected, and how the tool's outputs are presented to avoid confusion. You want quick, clear insights that support decisions without exposing patients to unnecessary risk.

Step 3: Design for reliability, training, and governance. Reliability means predictable performance, clear error handling, and robust uptime. Training involves teaching clinicians how to read AI outputs, when to trust them, and when to override. Governance covers how models are updated, how data quality is checked, and how you monitor for drift—when the tool's performance changes as data shifts over time. The best deployments build feedback loops so clinicians influence ongoing improvements.

Examples and micro-cases

Micro-case 1: A hospital adds an AI module to its PACS to pre-screen radiology images. Results appear next to each image with an easy-to-read color overlay. Radiologists receive a short briefing about potential findings, and a note automatically appears in the patient record. The workflow stays fast, and clinicians feel supported rather than slowed down.

Micro-case 2: A network of clinics tests an AI-assisted workflow for histopathology slides. Each lab adapts the tool to its stain types and scanner settings, with standardized checks to keep results consistent. Pathologists keep final say, but the AI's first pass saves time and helps catch subtle patterns.

Micro-case 3: An ophthalmology clinic uses AI to pre-screen fundus images before human review. The system flags urgent cases, so those patients are seen sooner. Clinicians report that reliance on the AI's triage reduces bottlenecks during screening campaigns.

Exercises

Exercise 1 (10 minutes): Review three sample AI outputs from imaging work. Note where the tool highlights regions, what the confidence scores suggest, and how you would respond in each case. Write down one question you would ask a colleague about each output.

Exercise 2 (15 minutes): Create a simple evaluation plan for a hypothetical imaging AI tool. List the data you would need, the metrics you would track, and how you would test generalization across hospitals. Include at least three checks you would perform before using it in patient care.

Exercise 3 (20 minutes): Map a small clinic's imaging workflow with an AI tool in mind. Draw or outline how images move from capture to review, where AI steps in, and where clinicians make the final call. Identify one potential bottleneck and one mitigation you would try.

Troubleshooting: quick fixes for common problems

- The AI misses certain findings on a new image type. Quick fix: gather more representative samples from that type and retrain or adjust the model with domain-specific features.

- Outputs are inconsistent across different scanners or sites. Quick fix: implement calibration steps and separate the model or layer weights by site, with standardized image preprocessing.

- Clinicians feel the AI adds steps rather than saves time. Quick fix: simplify the user interface, present results clearly in the same view as images, and provide short, targeted explanations of what the AI sees.

- Alerts cause alarm fatigue. Quick fix: tune thresholds to balance sensitivity and specificity and add a clinician override mechanism with a quick rationale entry.

- Data privacy concerns. Quick fix: ensure data handling follows privacy rules, use de-identified data for training when possible, and enable access controls and audit trails.

Tools and templates

- Quick evaluation checklist: Define task, gather data sources, select metrics, run external validation, compare to clinicians, set safety margins, document governance steps.

- Simple validation plan template: Problem description, data sources, data splits, metrics, expected outcomes, risk checks, sign-off steps.

- Deployment readiness sheet: PACS compatibility check, data flow diagram, access permissions, training plan, monitoring plan, escalation contacts.

Key Takeaway: AI image analysis works best when humans and machines cooperate, matching reliable outputs with clear clinical judgment and consistent workflows.

Coming up next: Subtittle: Natural Language Processing for Clinical Text

1) Extracting structured information from clinical notes, reports, and discharge summaries

2) Automatic documentation, summarization, and coding assistance

3) Handling clinical abbreviations, ambiguity, and multilingual corpora

Chapter 5

Natural Language Processing for Clinical Text

By the end of this chapter, you will understand how natural language processing helps unlock information from clinical text and support better care.

Step 1. Extracting structured information from clinical notes, reports, and discharge summaries

What you're learning here is how words in a note can become data you can act on. Clinicians write in freeform language, and a single note can hold a wealth of facts: diagnoses, medications, allergies, recent test results, and plans for the next steps. NLP helps take those unstructured words and turn them into structured pieces of information—little data packets that a computer can sort, compare, and use.

Think of a typical note. It mentions "the patient is started on lisinopril 5 mg daily," "history of type 2 diabetes," "no known drug allergies," and "follow-up in 2 weeks." An NLP approach will try to identify each of these items as discreet data points: medication name and dose, chronic condition, allergy status, and the timing of the follow-up. The value of doing this is clear: when data are structured, you can search across many notes quickly, flag important conditions, and build care plans that align with what the chart actually says.

Two essential ideas guide this step. First, you must locate the key phrases or entities that matter (medications, diagnoses, lab tests, dates, procedures) and recognize that different notes may call the same thing by different names. Second, you need to place those entities into a consistent format. For medications, that means standardizing the drug name, dosage, and route of administration. For diagnoses, it means mapping terms to a shared vocabulary or coding system so a “heart attack” and an "acute myocardial infarction" are treated as the same concept.

Two quick examples make this concrete. Example one: a progress note says "patient on amoxicillin 500 mg PO twice daily for 7 days." You would extract the drug name (amoxicillin), dose (500 mg), route (oral), frequency (twice daily), and duration (7 days). Example two: a discharge summary lists "A1c 7.8%, fasting glucose 128 mg/dL, no signs of nephropathy." You would pull out the biomarker (A1c), its value, and the accompanying interpretation about kidney health, so the chart reflects the patient's metabolic status without wading through narrative text.

In practice, you combine two kinds of approaches. Pattern-based rules can catch common phrases, while statistical models can learn from lots of notes to catch variations you might not anticipate. The goal isn't to replace clinicians' notes but to extend their usefulness by turning words into reliable data you can act on. With careful validation, you reduce manual re-entry, help clinicians see a patient's story at a glance, and improve consistency across the chart.

Step 2. Automatic documentation, summarization, and coding assistance

This step is about helping clinicians and health teams manage the sheer volume of writing that comes with care. NLP can draft concise summaries from longer notes, fill out routine documentation templates, and suggest codes for billing and data capture. When done thoughtfully, these tools save time and reduce fatigue, while still presenting human oversight so clinicians stay in control of what finally goes into the patient record.

Automatic documentation works best when it respects the clinical workflow. For example, after a patient visit, NLP can generate a draft discharge summary that hits the key points: reason for admission, major findings, tests performed, treatment given, and follow-up instructions. The clinician reviews and edits the draft, which is faster than starting from scratch. Such a workflow helps ensure that critical information isn't missed while keeping the clinician's voice intact in the final document.

Summarization is a cousin to documentation drafting. It condenses lengthy notes into short, readable paragraphs that highlight the essential facts. A well-crafted summary helps a busy clinician quickly grasp a patient's status during rounds or handoffs. It also benefits patients who want an accessible recap of their visit. The challenge is to preserve nuance—negations, risks, and the context of decision-making—so the summary remains accurate and useful.

Coding assistance ties NLP to administration and reimbursement. By suggesting potential codes based on the documented findings, NLP can speed up the coding process and improve consistency across encounters. The key is to avoid overreach: suggestions should be clearly labeled as provisional and always reviewed by a trained coder or clinician. When codes are accurate, administrative tasks become smoother, audits are easier, and the patient record reflects care more faithfully.

A pair of micro-cases helps illustrate this in action. Micro-case one: a clinician writes a short note after a procedure. NLP analyzes the text and suggests a matching set of CPT and ICD-10 codes, bundles the findings into a standard template, and produces a draft discharge instruction paragraph. The clinician then approves or adjusts, ensuring the final document is precise and complete. Micro-case two: a long history and examination note is transformed into a concise summary that emphasizes the diagnosis, major test results, planned interventions, and recommended follow-up, making it quicker for a clinician on the next shift to pick up where the last one left off.

The overarching idea is to use automation to handle repetitive writing tasks while preserving accuracy, clinician voice, and patient safety. When done well, documentation automation reduces time spent on clerical work and frees clinicians to focus more on direct patient care.

Step 3. Handling clinical abbreviations, ambiguity, and multilingual corpora

Notes are full of abbreviations like "MI," "BP," or "ECG," and the same terms can mean different things in different contexts. Abbreviations are shorthand for speed and clarity, but they also create risk if a system misreads them. Ambiguity arises when a term could point to more than one concept, depending on surrounding words, patient history, or the specialty involved. In multilingual settings, authors may switch between languages or mix terms, which adds another layer of complexity. NLP must handle all of this with sensitivity and accuracy.

One practical approach is to use context to disambiguate. For instance, the letters "MI" in a cardiology note are likely to mean myocardial infarction, while in a hardware or orthopedic note they might refer to mitral insufficiency or another term entirely. The surrounding sentences provide clues: patient age, referenced symptoms, recent imaging results, and the presence of procedure names can tilt interpretation in the right direction. A robust system also maintains a glossary of common abbreviations and preferred expansions to guide interpretation consistently.

Ambiguity can also be addressed by layering methods. Simple rules handle common, unambiguous patterns, while statistical methods —

trained on large, diverse data — learn to interpret more subtle cues. When notes are multilingual or include phrases in more than one language, a capable NLP system can switch models or apply translation-informed processing so that the same rules apply across languages. The goal is to preserve meaning and avoid misclassification that could change patient care down the line.

Two micro-cases illuminate this challenge. Micro-case one: a note states "BP 140/90," then later says "MI ruled out." The system needs to recognize that "BP" is blood pressure here, and ensure the blood pressure value is tied to the patient's vital signs rather than a diagnostic statement. Micro-case two: a bilingual chart includes "diabetes mellitus" alongside shorthand Spanish phrases like "hipertensión" (hypertension). A capable NLP pipeline recognizes the language switch and applies the same parsing logic across both languages, mapping terms to the same clinical concepts.

This trio of points—extracting structured data, automating documentation and coding, and managing abbreviations, ambiguity, and multilingual notes—gives you a practical toolkit. You learn not just to read words but to translate them into trustworthy, usable information. The aim is to support clinicians with reliable data, save time, and improve patient safety, all while keeping the human in the loop where it matters most.

Examples and micro-cases

Example 1: A clinician writes, "Patient denies chest pain. EKG normal. Lisinopril 10 mg daily continued." An NLP system flags the absence of chest pain (negation handling), records an ECG result as normal, and updates the medication list with the continued lisinopril dose. The outcome: a structured entry showing no chest pain, normal EKG, and active lisinopril therapy, ready for review.

Example 2: A discharge note reads, "Aspirin 81 mg, metformin 500 mg BID, and atorvastatin 20 mg QD prescribed." The NLP component extracts three medications, their doses, and frequencies and maps them to a standard medication list. It also verifies that the plan includes continued therapy and appropriate follow-up, which helps the next clinician understand the patient's baseline and treatment trajectory.

Exercises

1) Exercise: Practice two quick extractions on sample notes. Read a short note and identify at least five structured data points (medications, dosages, conditions, tests, dates). Time yourself for five minutes. Measure progress by listing each data point and noting how consistently you can map it to the same category across notes.

2) Exercise: Draft a one-paragraph automatic summary from a longer note. Use a provided sample note and write a concise summary that covers the reason for visit, key findings, plan, and follow-up. Spend about ten minutes. Check progress by asking a peer to read the summary and confirm that it captures the essential elements without adding new details.

3) Exercise: Create a mini-glossary of abbreviations you encounter in notes. List the abbreviation, what it most likely means in your setting, and an example sentence where it would be interpreted correctly. Do this in twenty minutes. Check progress by comparing your glossary with a

clinician's understanding of the most common terms in your notes.

4) Exercise: Test multilingual handling with a short bilingual note. If you have access to a sample that mixes languages, attempt to map terms to English equivalents and to the same clinical concepts. Time yourself for about 15 minutes. Measure progress by how many terms you can correctly map and whether the resulting structured data aligns with the narrative intent.

Troubleshooting

- Common problem: Negation misreads. Quick fix: verify negations with the surrounding sentence and, if possible, cross-check with explicit negation cues (no, denies, without). If misread, flag the data point for human review rather than using it as a trusted fact.

- Common problem: Abbreviation drift. Quick fix: maintain a living glossary and annotate uncertain expansions for review. When in doubt, defer to human confirmation.

- Common problem: Ambiguity in notes with multiple clinicians. Quick fix: seek consensus through a quick clinician check or rely on the most recent, most complete note to anchor interpretations.

- Common problem: Language mixing causing misinterpretation. Quick fix: apply language-detection steps and route notes to the appropriate language model; if necessary, flag for manual review when language boundaries are unclear.

Tools and templates

- Data extraction checklist: a short, repeatable checklist to identify medications, diagnoses, labs, dates, and procedures in notes.

- Abbreviation glossary template: a standard form with abbreviation, possible expansions, context cues, and confidence notes.

- Summary template: a concise two-to-three paragraph structure that covers reason for visit, key findings, plan, and follow-up.

- Coding suggestion sheet: a simple table mapping described findings to likely codes, with a column for clinician review.

- Example data map: a ready-to-use map that links extracted entities to a standardized terminology library for consistency.

Key Takeaway: Turning clinical text into reliable data helps clinicians act faster and safer, without losing the human touch.

Coming up next: Genomics, Precision Medicine, and Biomarker Discovery. AI approaches for variant interpretation and multi-omic integration, predictive models for treatment selection and patient stratification, and accelerating target identification and drug repurposing with computational screening. After you've learned how to read and summarize clinical text, you'll see how AI connects patient information to genetic data to personalize care.

Chapter 6

Genomics, Precision Medicine, and Biomarker Discovery

You are learning how AI helps unlock the power of genes, proteins, and medicines to tailor care. This chapter covers three big ideas: AI approaches for variant interpretation and multi-omic integration; predictive models for treatment selection and patient stratification; and speeding up target discovery and drug repurposing with computational screening.

1) AI approaches for variant interpretation and multi-omic integration

Step 1: Define the problem and gather data

You start by asking: Which genetic variants might matter for a patient's health, and what other data can help clarify their role? You look for two kinds of information: (a) genetic variants found in the genome, and (b) other layers of biology that show how the body works, like how genes are turned into proteins, how proteins interact, and how small molecules affect the system. The goal is to connect a genetic signal to a potential health effect, while recognizing uncertainty. The data you use should be as complete and clean as possible, and you should respect privacy and consent rules as you gather it. The idea is not to prove a diagnosis with a single data point, but to build a clearer, probabilistic picture by layering information.

Step 2: Use AI to interpret variants and connect to other omics

AI helps by taking many small clues—from a DNA change, to how a gene is expressed in a tissue, to how a protein behaves—and combining them to estimate the likely impact of that variant. The approach is not to replace knowledge about biology, but to extend it, using patterns learned from large datasets. You can think of it as a smart aggregator: it weighs conservation across species, known disease associations, tissue-specific activity, and how a variant might alter protein function or splicing. When you bring in multi-omic data—gene expression, protein levels, metabolic signals—the AI system can spot connections that aren't obvious from one dataset alone. This helps prioritize which variants deserve deeper study and how they might contribute to a patient's condition.

Example 1 (micro-case): In a fictional dataset, you find a rare change in a gene linked to metabolism. Alone, the variant is unclear. When you add expression data showing high activity of that gene in liver tissue and a related protein's behavior in metabolism, the AI tool notes a higher probability that this variant could affect metabolic pathways. The result is a ranked list of variants to review, with a short note about how they might influence disease risk in the liver.

Example 2 (micro-case): A patient's data include genomics plus transcriptomics (RNA) data. The AI system looks for patterns that tie a variant to altered gene expression in a disease-relevant tissue and to changes in a connected network of proteins. It flags a plausible pathway change and suggests a possible biomarker to watch, even when the variant's effect isn't fully proven yet. The clinician can then decide whether to pursue further testing or monitoring.

A practical workflow you can follow begins with collecting clean basic data, then layering in omics information, and finally letting AI highlight the most informative signals. The key is to treat AI as a guide that helps you sort through many hints, not as a sole decision-maker. You should always bring clinical judgment, patient context, and ethics into every interpretation.

2) Predictive models for treatment selection and patient stratification

Step 3: Gather clinical and omic features, then choose a model that fits the task

You assemble a set of features that might influence treatment choices: disease type, stage, patient age, and relevant omics data such as genomic variants, expression patterns, or protein markers. You then pick a modeling approach that balances accuracy with interpretability. For clinicians and patients, understanding why a model suggests a treatment matters as much as how good the prediction is. So you favor models that can explain their main drivers, even if they are simpler. You also plan for how to test the model on new patients to see if it holds up outside the data you trained on.

Step 4: Validate the model, check fairness, and interpret outputs

Validation means testing the model on data it hasn't seen yet and checking how well its predictions match real outcomes. You look for reasonable accuracy and useful distinctions between patient groups. Fairness matters: you check whether the model's performance is similar across ages, genders, ethnic backgrounds, and other patient subgroups. If you find gaps, you adjust the model or add more diverse data. Then you translate the model's outputs into actionable guidance: which patients might benefit from a certain therapy, what level of confidence to place in the prediction, and what monitoring should follow. The aim is to give clinicians a practical tool that improves decision-making while avoiding risky overinterpretation.

Example 3 (micro-case): In a small, imagined study, you combine patient age, disease stage, and a multi-omics profile to predict who will respond best to a new targeted therapy. The model shows that younger patients with a particular expression pattern have higher response rates, but it also notes some uncertainty. You view this as a guide rather than a decree, using it to discuss options with the patient and to plan follow-up tests that can confirm or challenge the prediction.

Example 4 (micro-case): A hospital cohort includes patients with the same disease but different genetic backgrounds. A fairness check shows the model performs a bit better for one demographic. You address this by gathering more diverse data, adjusting the model, and communicating the limits clearly to the care team. The result is a more reliable tool for guiding treatment choices across a broader patient group.

Think of predictive models as decision support that helps you identify who might benefit from a therapy, what risks to monitor, and where to focus resources for the best outcomes. They don't replace clinical judgment, but they can sharpen it by surfacing patterns that are hard to see from a single data source.

3) Accelerating target identification and drug repurposing with computational screening

Step 5: Identify targets using computational methods

For many diseases, the goal is to find a target that, when modulated, can improve outcomes. AI and computation help by mapping disease biology to networks of genes, proteins, and pathways. You look for points in the network where a change could have a meaningful effect, while trying to avoid targets that could cause too many side effects. This work often uses existing knowledge about pathways, structural data about proteins, and models of how different molecules interact. The point is to narrow down the field to the most promising ideas so scientists can test them more efficiently in the lab and clinic.

Step 6: Screen existing drugs for repurposing and consider safety

Drug repurposing uses existing medicines in new ways. Computational screening compares drug signatures (how a drug affects biology) with disease signatures (how a disease changes biology) to spot good matches. The advantage is speed and safety: these drugs have already been studied for safety in people, which can shorten the path to use in new conditions. You always consider safety, interactions with other medicines, and patient context before any real-world application. In silico screening is a powerful first pass that helps researchers decide which drugs deserve laboratory and clinical testing.

Example 5 (micro-case): Researchers assemble a disease signature from gene expression changes and compare it to signatures produced by hundreds of approved drugs. They find a commonly used medication that could modulate a key pathway involved in the disease. Early lab tests show the drug affects the pathway as predicted, which prompts a small, careful clinical exploration with close monitoring.

Example 6 (micro-case): A team uses a network model to identify a protein that sits at a hub of several disease-related pathways. They run a virtual screen to see which approved drugs might interact with that protein. They find a drug with a known safety profile that could influence multiple steps in the disease process. This finding doesn't prove the drug works for the condition, but it gives researchers a concrete, testable lead.

In this part of the field, the goal is to move from a big map of biology to a short list of testable ideas. You start with wide exploration, then narrow to a few promising targets or drugs, and finally confirm with lab experiments and carefully designed clinical studies. AI helps you see what to test first, but you still need careful validation and patient-centered considerations every step of the way.

Exercises

1) Variant interpretation plan (20 minutes). Write down a simple plan that lists the variant types you would investigate, the data you would collect, and the basic AI tools you would use to weigh evidence. Measure progress by having a peer review your plan for clarity and realism.

2) Mini multi-omics integration sketch (15–25 minutes). Draw a small map showing how genomics, transcriptomics, and proteomics could be connected for a hypothetical patient. Note at least two links between data layers and one potential pitfall. Measure progress by explaining your map aloud to a friend or colleague.

3) Model sanity check and interpretation (20–30 minutes). Create a one-page outline for a simple predictive model: which features you would include, what outcome you would predict, and how you would check fairness. Measure progress by verifying that the plan includes a validation step and a plan for addressing bias.

4) Drug repurposing drill (15–25 minutes). In a simple scenario, pick three drugs and describe, at a high level, how their known actions could relate to a hypothetical disease's biology. Note safety considerations and what would be required to test these ideas further. Measure progress by summarizing your three picks and the next steps you would take.

Troubleshooting: Quick fixes for common obstacles

- If data are incomplete or biased, you get unreliable predictions. Fix by identifying missing data, diversifying sources, and clearly labeling uncertainty in outputs.

- If a model is hard to interpret, choose simpler models or add explanations for the main drivers. Keep the clinician's perspective in mind when presenting results.

- If results vary across patient groups, stop and re-check data quality, expand the dataset, or adjust the model to reduce bias. Document what you change and why.

- If a target or drug suggestion seems biologically vague, return to the underlying biology, add more context from known pathways, and seek expert review before proceeding to lab tests.

Tools and templates you can copy

- Variant interpretation checklist: Data quality check, variant annotation, predicted impact, tissue relevance, uncertainty notes, next steps.

- Multi-omics integration plan: List of omics data for this use case, linking rules between layers, expected added value, validation plan.

- Predictive model brief: Target outcome, features to include, simple model type, validation approach, fairness checks, how results will be communicated to clinicians.

- Target discovery brief: Disease biology summary, candidate pathways, network hubs to explore, criteria to deem a target promising, plan for experimental validation.

- Drug repurposing plan: Disease signature, drug signature databases, scoring rubric for matches, safety and interaction considerations, plan for lab tests.

Key Takeaway: AI helps connect genetic signals to real-world biology by layering data and patterns, but human judgment, patient context, and careful validation are essential before using any result in care.

Coming up next Subtittle: Decision Support and Treatment Optimization

1) Design of point-of-care decision support tools and alerting systems,

2) Personalized dosing, therapy recommendations, and outcome prediction,

3) Closed-loop systems for monitoring and adapting treatment over time

Chapter 7

Decision Support and Treatment Optimization

By the end of this chapter, you will know how to design point-of-care decision support tools, personalize treatment decisions safely, and describe how closed-loop monitoring can adapt care over time.

Design of point-of-care decision support tools and alerting systems

You want tools that help clinicians make better, faster decisions without getting in the way. Start by clarifying who will use the tool and what success looks like. Talk with doctors, nurses, pharmacists, and other care team members. Agree on clear goals, such as reducing missed warnings, improving response times, or catching dangerous drug interactions early. Define simple success metrics you can track: alert accuracy, time saved per shift, and the rate at which recommendations are followed. If you start with vague aims, you'll build a tool that pleases no one and risks adding work rather than reducing it.

Next, map how data will flow. Identify the sources you will connect to—electronic health records, vitals, lab results, imaging reports, and medication lists—and decide how the tool will present information. Design your interface to be unobtrusive. Clinicians should see a concise alert or recommendation within their ordinary workflow, not in a separate portal. Use intuitive language, avoid jargon, and present the most urgent items first. Build in a way to filter or tailor alerts by setting severity levels and allowing clinicians to adjust sensitivity within safe bounds. This reduces noise and keeps attention where it matters.

Then define the decision logic and alert criteria. Create rules that translate patient data into concrete recommendations or warnings. Use straightforward thresholds or, when possible, evidence-based patterns that have broad, general support. The logic should be explainable: the clinician should be able to see why an alert fired and what action is suggested. Include a concise rationale and a recommended action, not a long research summary. Design the system to allow clinicians to provide feedback on alerts, so the tool can learn what works in real settings and what doesn't.

Plan for alert fatigue and workload. Alerts are powerful, but too many can overwhelm. Build safety features: tiered alerts, the option to acknowledge and document, and a default path that requires human confirmation before a major change. Include an easy “snooze” or “dismiss with reason” function for non-urgent items. Regularly review false positives and adjust your criteria to maintain trust. When clinicians trust the alerts, they use them as intended and the entire care process improves.

Pilot the tool in a low-risk setting first. Use a small unit, a specific patient group, or a single workflow to test whether the design fits real practice. Collect feedback after shifts, not just after a month. Observe how clinicians interact with the tool, what alerts they act on, and where friction appears. Use these observations to refine the interface, thresholds, and reminder cadence before expanding.

Examples and micro-cases. In one hospital unit, an alert analyzes vitals trends and lab data to flag potential sepsis early in the emergency department. A nurse sees a short, clear notification with three recommended actions: obtain a blood culture, start a broad-spectrum antibiotic according to local guidelines, and monitor the patient every hour. In a clinic, an alert notifies the clinician if a newly prescribed medication could interact with a current drug list, offering a safe alternative and a brief justification. In both cases, the tool supports the clinician, but the final decision remains with the human expert.

Personalized dosing, therapy recommendations, and outcome prediction

Personalized care starts with the idea that not all patients respond the same way to a medication or a plan. The goal is reasonable: tailor dosing and treatment choices to improve the likelihood of good outcomes while reducing risk. Start by identifying the patient outcomes you want to influence. For many conditions, this could mean achieving target blood levels, reducing symptom scores, or shortening hospital stays. Keep expectations realistic and communicate uncertainty clearly. A good dosing or therapy recommendation should support the clinician's judgment, not replace it.

Gather the right data. Collect relevant patient information such as age, weight, organ function markers, prior responses to treatment, comorbidities, and important lifestyle factors. You don't need every data point in the world; you need the ones that most strongly influence the outcome you aim to predict. If some data are missing or delayed, have a plan to handle that gracefully, such as using recent values and clearly indicating when a recommendation is based on partial information. The idea is to make the system robust enough to work in real hospital settings with imperfect data.

Choose an appropriate approach. You can use simple rule-based logic—like adjusting a dose based on a patient's kidney function—or more flexible models that learn from patterns in large patient groups. If you use learning models, ensure they are transparent enough to explain why a suggestion was made. Explainability matters in medicine: clinicians should be able to see the factors behind a recommendation and the confidence level, not just a single number.

Integrate with the clinical workflow. A dosing or treatment recommendation should appear where clinicians already spend their time, such as during order entry or in the patient's chart review. Provide a brief, actionable suggestion and a short note on why it's reasonable, plus any safety cautions. Allow clinicians to adjust the recommendation, add notes, or request a second opinion within the same screen.

The system should not force a choice or interrupt critical processes without a clear, justified reason.

Validate with data and real roles. Start with retrospective validation on past cases to see if the recommendations align with what clinicians did and what led to better outcomes. Then run small-scale pilot tests with real patients under careful supervision. Track how often clinicians use the recommendations, how often those outcomes improve, and whether any new risks appear. Validation is not a one-time task; it's an ongoing activity that keeps the system trustworthy.

Communicate uncertainty and provide alternatives. Medicine is rarely certain. When a prediction has a margin of error, say so plainly and present a few reasonable options rather than a single "correct" answer. This helps clinicians balance data-driven guidance with their experience and patient preferences. Include optional notes for the patient or family if appropriate, helping everyone understand the plan.

Examples and micro-cases. In diabetes care, a dosing recommendation might adjust insulin by small, safe increments based on recent glucose readings, activity level, and meals, with a clear range and a caution about hypoglycemia. In oncology, a therapy recommendation could weigh expected benefit against toxicity risk, offering a preferred option plus a secondary choice and a brief rationale. In antibiotic stewardship, a clinician could see a suggested duration based on infection type and local resistance data, with a note about when to reassess.

What makes a good personalized recommendation? It is grounded in patient data, easy to review, and adaptable. It respects clinical judgment and clarifies why a suggestion makes sense. It also avoids forcing a single path; instead, it provides a smart starting point and a safe space to adjust as needed. When clinicians trust the recommendations, they can tailor care without being pushed into a rigid protocol.

Closed-loop systems for monitoring and adapting treatment over time

A closed-loop system continuously monitors a patient and adjusts treatment in response to what happens next. The aim is smoother care, fewer delays, and the ability to respond to changing conditions without waiting for a clinician to intervene every time. A practical closed-loop system has three core elements: safe monitoring, reliable feedback, and a clear, human-in-the-loop safeguard.

Define what you will monitor and establish safety boundaries. Choose measurable indicators that reflect the treatment's effect and patient safety, such as vital signs, lab values, or treatment response markers. Set upper and lower safety limits and decide what constitutes a meaningful change versus a temporary fluctuation. Clear limits prevent the system from making risky adjustments and make it easier to recognize when something is off track.

Create a safe feedback mechanism. The system should be able to adjust therapy within a predefined safe range and automatically flag potential problems for clinician review if the change could be risky. The feedback loop must be transparent:

clinicians should see what was adjusted, why, and what the expected outcome is. Provide an option to pause automatic changes and require human confirmation if the situation is uncertain or if the patient's condition worsens.

Ensure human oversight and accountability. Even a well-designed closed-loop system needs a human in the loop. Clinicians should be able to review all adjustments, revert changes if needed, and document decisions in the patient's record. Build in fail-safes: if data quality deteriorates, if alerts exceed a threshold, or if the patient's condition changes rapidly, the system should revert to manual control or escalate appropriately.

Test gradually in controlled settings. Begin with simulations and then move to small, carefully monitored pilots. Track safety events, time to intervention, and patient outcomes to determine whether the closed loop adds value without introducing new risks. If the system behaves differently in real life than in simulations, adjust its rules and safety checks accordingly.

Examples and micro-cases. In a hospital ICU, a closed-loop system might monitor a patient's blood pressure, heart rate, and medication levels and adjust a vasopressor dose within a safe range. If the patient starts to deteriorate, the system flags the change and requires clinician review before continuing. In a long-term care setting, a system could adjust fluid or electrolyte management in response to trending labs, with regular reminders for clinician checks.

Troubleshooting and practical notes

Common problems include alert fatigue, data gaps, and mismatches between the tool's recommendations and local practice. If clinicians ignore alerts, revisit alert criteria for redundancy or non-urgent items. If data are missing or delayed, add fallback rules and explain when a recommendation is based on partial information. If workflow clashes reduce use, redesign the interface to align with existing clinician routines and ensure the tool never blocks critical tasks.

A few quick fixes you can apply now:

Reassess alert thresholds after a two-week pilot to reduce non-essential alerts.

Add a brief, patient-specific note that explains why a recommendation matters.

Provide a one-click exit path for any automated action, with a clear reason recorded.

Label data provenance (where data came from and when) so clinicians trust the source.

Regularly collect user feedback and schedule monthly reviews of performance metrics.

Templates and tools you can copy

Decision-support design checklist: clarifies the user, objective, data sources, and success metrics; includes a safety review step.

Alert criteria template: captures the alert name, trigger data, severity level, action recommended, and理由 (brief justification) to help explain decisions to users.

Dosing decision note template: a compact note that accompanies each recommendation, listing patient factors, suggested dose range, safety reminders, and monitoring plan.

Workflow integration map: a simple schematic that shows where the decision-support tool fits into the clinician's normal steps, where alerts appear, and what actions are allowed.

Validation plan outline: a lightweight plan that lists retrospective checks, pilot goals, and metrics to track in the first real-world test.

Exercises

1. Interview two clinicians about what information they need most at the point of care. Time: 15 minutes. Outcome: a prioritized list of needs.

2. Sketch a screen showing an alert arriving in a clinician's workflow. Time: 20 minutes. Outcome: a draft layout focusing on clarity and minimal disruption.

3. Map data sources for a common condition you've studied. Time: 25 minutes. Outcome: a data-source map with data owners and update frequencies.

4. Describe a decision-rule you would implement in a simple CDS tool. Time: 15 minutes. Outcome: a concrete rule and its expected impact.

5. Write a short rationale for a two-sentence alert message. Time: 10 minutes. Outcome: an explainable justification that fits on one screen.

6. Create a plan to test an alert with a two-week pilot. Time: 30 minutes. Outcome: a pilot protocol and safety checks.

7. List three potential sources of false positives in your setting. Time: 15 minutes. Outcome: a mitigation plan for each source.

8. Propose how to handle data delays in decision support. Time: 15 minutes. Outcome: a fallback strategy that keeps the workflow moving.

9. Draft a one-page user guide for clinicians. Time: 60 minutes. Outcome: a concise, usable reference.

10. Run a mini-review of a dosing guideline and translate it into a simple recommendation. Time: 30 minutes. Outcome: a practical dosing suggestion.

11. Create a simple confidence indicator for a recommendation. Time: 20 minutes. Outcome: a three-tier confidence view (low, medium, high).

12. Design a safety pause option for automatic changes. Time: 20 minutes. Outcome: a one-click manual override flow.

13. List at least five patient factors to include in a personalization rule. Time: 20 minutes. Outcome: a factor checklist.

14. Draft a short clinical note explaining an automated action after an adjustment. Time: 15

minutes. Outcome: a clear documentation template.

15. Prepare a two-page comparison of rule-based vs. model-based recommendations. Time: 40 minutes. Outcome: a balanced view of trade-offs.

16. Outline how you would validate a new decision tool using retrospective data. Time: 45 minutes. Outcome: a validation plan with metrics.

17. Create a simple patient example showing how a personalized dosing decision could unfold. Time: 30 minutes. Outcome: a micro-case narrative.

18. Draft a nurse-friendly version of an alert description. Time: 25 minutes. Outcome: an accessible message for non-physician users.

19. List potential privacy and security concerns for decision support. Time: 20 minutes. Outcome: a risk list with mitigations.

20. Draft a short incident report template for when a decision-support action goes wrong. Time: 15 minutes. Outcome: a usable report form.

21. Design a quick-check checklist to verify data quality before an alert fires. Time: 20 minutes. Outcome: a ready-to-use checklist.

22. Create a one-page guide to interpret a simple outcome prediction. Time: 15 minutes. Outcome: a lay explanation with a confidence note.

23. Develop a small workflow demonstration you could run with a colleague. Time: 30 minutes. Outcome: a hands-on practice session.

24. Prepare a brief consensus note for a team meeting about adopting decision-support tools. Time: 20 minutes. Outcome: a presentation-ready summary.

Troubleshooting quick fixes

If results vary by department, adjust the rules to fit local practice and user feedback. If users report too many alerts, reduce non-critical items and increase the threshold for urgency. If the tool's recommendations feel unfamiliar, add concise explanations and keep the language plain. If data quality is inconsistent, implement clear data provenance notes and emphasize what the tool can still do with partial information. If clinicians hesitate to use the tool, run short, supervised practice sessions and invite early adopters to share how the tool helps in real cases.

Coming up next Subtittle: From Prototype to Practice: Implementation Strategies

1) Designing pilots, clinical trials, and real-world validation studies,

2) Workflow redesign, clinician training, and change management tactics,

3) Operationalizing deployment: infrastructure, scaling, and reliability engineering

Chapter 8

From Prototype to Practice: Implementation Strategies

You will be able to design pilots, streamline workflows, and prepare for deployment of AI in healthcare with confidence.

Point 1: Designing pilots, clinical trials, and real-world validation studies

When you start turning an AI idea into practice, you need a clear map for testing. Your first goal is to prove that the tool helps in real settings and stays safe for patients. Begin by naming the problem you're solving and deciding how you'll know if you've solved it. You should set concrete success metrics that matter to clinicians and patients. For example, you might measure whether the AI reduces time to decision, improves accuracy of a diagnosis, or lowers unnecessary tests. Decide what counts as a win and how you'll recognize it.

Next, pick the kind of test that fits your situation. A pilot in one department can be very different from a broader trial across multiple sites. A pilot often stays small and tightly controlled, with close supervision and careful data collection. A real-world validation study looks at how the tool performs in everyday work, across diverse patients and workflows. The choice depends on the risk level of the tool, the data you have, and the readiness of your system. The important thing is to set boundaries: what will be measured, what outcomes you will monitor, and how you'll react if things don't go as planned.

Finally, plan the path from test to trust. You want a plan for both the clinical trial style phase and the real-world validation phase. In the trial phase, you outline eligibility, endpoints, consent, data handling, and oversight. In real-world validation, you describe how you'll monitor performance in routine care, collect feedback from clinicians, and verify that safety remains intact during everyday use. You'll also want a simple governance framework that covers data privacy, risk management, and rapid stop rules if patient safety or accuracy dips.

Example 1: Radiology triage tool in an emergency department

You start by defining the problem: triage decisions should be faster and as accurate as possible. You set metrics: time to initial triage decision, rate of missed critical findings, and clinician satisfaction with the tool. In a controlled pilot, you pair the AI with a small group of radiologists and test on a subset of cases during a shift. You collect data on performance, but you keep human review for flagged cases. After a few weeks, you expand to a second department to compare settings and adjust thresholds. The goal is to show that the tool helps, without increasing risk, before broader use.

Example 2: EHR note summarizer for post-visit summaries

You outline that the summarizer should produce concise notes that travelers through the chart meet certain length and clarity standards. In the first phase, you run the tool on retrospective notes to check coverage and coherence. In the live pilot, clinicians review and correct a portion of summaries, and you track how often the AI saves time while preserving essential details. This approach helps you learn where the AI shines and where human review remains essential.

Two practical micro-exercises to anchor this point:

- Exercise A: Write your pilot objective and success metrics in one page. Time yourself for 25 minutes. Outcome: a crisp objective and a list of 3–5 measurable results you'll watch.

- Exercise B: Sketch a pilot plan in simple steps for your setting. Include setting, participants, data you'll collect, duration, and decision rules. Timebox to 30 minutes. Outcome: a draft plan you can share with a supervisor for feedback.

- Exercise C: Draft a basic governance outline. List who reviews risk, what data you'll protect, and when you'll pause the pilot. Time: 20 minutes. Outcome: a simple risk-and-go/no-go framework.

Troubleshooting for this first area

- If stakeholders keep shifting metrics, return to a single, prioritized objective and re-align the plan. Quick fix: agree on one primary endpoint and two secondary ones, then document decisions.

- If data quality stalls progress, pause to fix data collection rules and annotation standards. A minimal data-quality checklist helps keep the pilot moving.

- If you encounter regulatory ambiguity, document the questions and escalate to a governance body to decide how to proceed, even if answers come later.

Tools and templates to support this point

- Pilot objective and metrics template: a one-page form to capture problem, success metrics, and decision rules.

- Pilot plan checklist: setting, scope, data, roles, duration, and stop rules.

- Validation plan skeleton: endpoints, methods, data capture, and oversight steps.

Point 2: Workflow redesign, clinician training, and change management tactics

A tool can fail if it doesn't fit into how people actually work. Your job is to redesign workflows so the AI complements clinicians, not complicates their day. Start by mapping the current workflow end-to-end. Where do tasks slow down? Where do errors tend to happen? That map will reveal the places where AI can help, such as reducing repetitive data entry, prioritizing cases, or highlighting relevant information. The aim is to preserve essential elements of clinical judgment while removing unnecessary friction.

With the map in hand, design AI-augmented workflows. This means specifying when the AI should act, what it should present, and how clinicians should respond. For example, should the AI provide a short note, a flag, or a recommended course of action? Decide how it appears in the user interface, how it integrates with existing systems, and how you'll handle exceptions. Involve frontline clinicians in this design so the tool feels familiar and useful, not alien.

The heart of change management is training and ongoing support. Build a simple training program that teaches users how to interact with the tool, what the outputs mean, and how to handle uncertainties. Offer hands-on practice, quick-reference guides, and an easy way to report problems. Create a feedback loop where clinicians can share what works, what doesn't, and what improvements they want next. Monitor adoption, celebrate early wins, and adjust your approach as needed.

Two micro-cases illustrating this point

- Case A: Workflow for a decision-support alert in primary care

Before: clinicians juggle lab results, notes, and patient history in multiple screens. After: an alert flags a critical lab abnormality with a short rationale and a one-click recommended action. Clinicians report faster decisions and fewer missed abnormalities in week-to-week comparisons.

- Case B: AI-assisted documentation in postoperative rounds

Before: clinicians spend many minutes typing notes. After: the AI suggests a concise note outline and fills in standard phrases. Clinicians save time and quality remains high, with a check on the AI-generated text for accuracy.

Two practical exercises for this point

- Exercise D: Create a one-page workflow map for your setting, marking where AI could help and where it should not intervene. Time: 40 minutes. Outcome: a clear map with at least two AI touchpoints.

- Exercise E: Draft a clinician training plan for the AI tool. Include a short training session, a quick-reference guide, and a feedback channel. Time: 45 minutes. Outcome: a ready-to-run training plan that supports adoption.

- Exercise F: Build a simple change-management plan that includes milestones, champions, and communication steps. Time: 30 minutes. Outcome: a plan that keeps people engaged during rollout.

Troubleshooting for this point

- If adoption stalls, identify a single "champion" in each clinical area to model usage and gather feedback. Quick fix: set up weekly short coaching sessions.

- If the tool feels intrusive, revise when and how alerts appear, and ensure clinicians can customize thresholds or disable features without penalty.

- If training doesn't translate to use, shorten training modules, add hands-on practice, and ensure easy access to help and examples.

Tools and templates to support this point

- Workflow mapping template: steps, decision points, AI touchpoints, and owner responsibilities.

- Clinician training plan template: goals, modules, practice time, and feedback loops.

- Change-management checklist: stakeholder engagement, comms plan, milestones, and champions network.

Point 3: Operationalizing deployment: infrastructure, scaling, and reliability engineering

Pulling it all together means making sure the technical backbone and processes can support dependable AI in everyday care. Start with a practical infrastructure plan that respects data security, system reliability, and easy maintenance. You need to specify where data lives, who can access it, how updates roll out, and how you will protect patient privacy. Your plan should also include a roadmap for scaling: how the system expands from a single department to a hospital network, and how performance benchmarks travel with scale.

Next, turn the plan into dependable operations. Reliability engineering means you build monitoring into the deployment from day one. Set up dashboards that track key performance indicators, such as latency, uptime, and error rates. Establish incident response playbooks so your team knows what to do if something goes wrong—who to alert, how to rollback, and how to communicate with clinicians and patients. You should also design a simple update process. AI models evolve; you need a safe way to retrain, validate, and deploy improvements without disrupting care.

Finally, consider scaling and governance hand-in-hand. As you grow, you must maintain data governance, security, and privacy standards. Create a lightweight risk register that your team reviews regularly. Ensure that audits, provenance, and traceability are built into the deployment so you can explain decisions and outcomes if questions arise. A practical deployment plan also calls for reliability engineering principles like redundancy, backups, and disaster recovery rehearsals.

Two micro-cases to illustrate deployment in action

- Case C: A hospital-wide deployment of a lab-result triage AI

You begin with a single unit, then extend to multiple departments. You monitor latency, false positives, and clinician feedback. When the tool proves stable, you scale gradually with robust change management and a clear rollback path.

- Case D: A cloud-based decision-support tool for oncology clinics

You start with a careful data governance plan, ensure secure access, and implement a staged rollout. You monitor performance across sites, and you have a clear plan for updates that keeps care uninterrupted.

Three practical exercises for this point

- Exercise G: Draft a deployment infrastructure map. Identify data location, access controls, and update pathways. Time: 40 minutes. Outcome: a clear diagram and policy notes.

- Exercise H: Create a reliability and monitoring plan. List what you will monitor, how you will respond to incidents, and who is in charge. Time: 40 minutes. Outcome: an active monitoring plan.

- Exercise I: Prepare a scaling plan with milestones and risk checks. Time: 30 minutes. Outcome: a staged growth plan with clear checkpoints.

Troubleshooting for deployment

- If the system is slow or unresponsive, investigate bottlenecks in data flow or server capacity. Quick fix: scale up resources during peak times or optimize data pipelines.

- If updates cause issues in care workflows, implement a blue-green deployment approach so you can switch back quickly if needed.

- If security or privacy worries surface, revisit access controls, auditing, and encryption practices. Bring governance teams into the loop and tighten checks.

Tools and templates to support this point

- Deployment readiness checklist: hardware, software, data, security, and personnel readiness.

- Monitoring dashboard template: key metrics to track, with thresholds and escalation paths.

- Incidence response playbook: steps to detect, diagnose, and recover from failures.

Coming up next: Ethics, Regulation, and Risk Management

1) Mitigating bias, ensuring equity, and conducting fairness audits

2) Regulatory pathways, certification standards, and compliance requirements

3) Liability, informed consent, and patient autonomy in AI-enabled care

Key Takeaway: You can design, test, and deploy AI in healthcare in a way that builds real-world value while safeguarding patients, by tying pilots to clear metrics, aligning workflows with clinical practice, and making reliability a central habit.

Coming up next: In the next chapter, you'll explore ethics, regulation, and risk management more deeply, learning how to spot bias, navigate certification, and protect patient autonomy in AI-enabled care.

Chapter 9

Ethics, Regulation, and Risk Management

You will learn to navigate ethics, regulation, and risk in AI-enabled healthcare to build fair, compliant tools that protect patients.

Mitigating bias, ensuring equity, and conducting fairness audits

Bias can sneak into AI in quiet, everyday ways. It can show up in the data you train on, the people who design and test the system, or in how the tool is used in real clinics. When data reflect only a narrow group, the model may perform well for that group but poorly for others. When designers assume what patients need without asking, the tool may push decisions that aren't best for everyone. The goal is to see those blind spots before they cause harm and to fix them as you go.

Step 1: Audit your data for representativeness. Look at who is included in your data and who isn't. Are there gaps in age, gender, ethnicity, location, or disease stage? If you find gaps, plan to fill them with additional data or design choices that reduce reliance on limited samples. The principle is simple: data should reflect the real world where the tool will operate, not just the subset you happened to collect.

Step 2: Define fairness goals and metrics early. Decide which groups you want to compare and what counts as acceptable performance. Common ideas include equal accuracy across groups or similar error rates across populations. The key is to be explicit about what fairness means for your tool and your patients, and to document those definitions so everyone knows what you're aiming for.

Step 3: Create diverse validation and test sets. When you test, use data slices that represent different populations, settings, and scenarios. Don't rely on a single overall score. Break out results by subgroup and by real-world context, such as different clinics or patient languages. The rationale is that a good tool should perform well across the people it will serve, not just on average.

Step 4: Run controlled experiments to assess impact across groups. If a change improves performance for one group but hurts another, you need to understand why and adjust. This is a practical moment to balance benefits while protecting against unintended harms. The aim is to avoid deploying a tool that benefits some patients while harming others.

Step 5: Document limitations and remediation plans. Keep an audit trail that explains where bias was detected, what was done to fix it, and what remains uncertain. This record helps teams learn, satisfies regulators and auditors, and builds trust with clinicians and patients.

Step 6: Establish ongoing governance and stakeholder involvement. Create a standing group that includes clinicians, patients, ethicists, and data experts who review fairness issues, performance drift, and updates. Fairness is not a one-time check;

it's an ongoing practice that happens as data change and as you deploy in new places.

Two brief micro-cases to illustrate

First, imagine a computer-aided imaging tool trained mostly on adult male patients. In a fairness audit, you notice that accuracy for detecting a common condition in women is significantly lower. You respond by gathering more images from women, adjusting the model, and validating again across both groups. After retraining, the tool becomes steadier for everyone, with more consistent results across sexes.

Second, think of an NLP tool that helps extract symptoms from discharge notes in several languages. If the tool is better at English notes than notes written in a regional language, you may see systematic gaps. You address this by adding language-specific samples, tuning language models for those dialects, and validating with clinicians who speak those languages. The outcome is clearer, more reliable documentation across diverse patients.

Regulatory pathways, certification standards, and compliance requirements

Healthcare AI sits at the crossroads of medicine, safety, privacy, and patient trust. Regulators set expectations for safety, effectiveness, reliability, and data protection. Rules vary by country and often depend on how a tool is used in practice—whether it's a decision support aid, a diagnosis tool, or an automated process that affects treatment. The broad idea is that you must prove your tool helps patients without causing new risks, and you must protect patient information every step of the way.

Step 1: Identify the regulatory category and applicable rules. Start by asking: In my country, is this software considered medical device software, a clinical decision support system, or something else? The answer shapes what evidence you need and which approvals you might seek. Laws often require systematic risk assessments, quality management practices, and clear documentation.

Step 2: Plan for safety risk management and quality systems. Build a process to identify hazards, evaluate how severe and likely they are, and decide how to reduce risk. Establish a quality system that covers development, testing, deployment, maintenance, and change control. The idea is to create a reliable, repeatable path from concept to clinic.

Step 3: Gather evidence for validation. You'll usually prepare three kinds of validation: analytical (does the tool do what it says it should under controlled conditions), clinical (does it help patients in real care settings), and usability (is it easy for clinicians to use correctly). Collect data, run tests, and document results clearly. The purpose is to show the tool is safe, useful, and reliable in practice.

Step 4: Ensure data privacy and security. Protect patient information by using solid data governance, access controls, encryption, and audit logs. Policies should explain who can see what data, how data is stored, and what happens if a breach occurs. Privacy protection isn't just a box to check—it's essential to keeping patients confident in AI-enabled care.

Step 5: Seek appropriate certification or regulatory endorsement when needed. Some tools require formal recognition or registration before they can be marketed or used widely. The exact path can vary, but the principle is the same: make sure the tool has gone through the right gates so clinicians and patients can trust it.

Step 6: Maintain ongoing compliance and reporting. Regulations can evolve as new technologies emerge. You should monitor changes, update risk assessments, refresh validation studies, and keep transparency with patients and clinicians about any changes that could affect safety or performance.

Two micro-cases to illustrate

Consider a hospital deploying a new AI tool to help with imaging triage. The team begins with a regulatory assessment to determine whether clinical trials are needed and which certifications would apply in their jurisdiction. They gather validation data from multiple sites, ensure data privacy protections, and prepare documents showing how they monitor performance after deployment. The tool receives the necessary clearance, and clinicians feel confident using it as a support, not a replacement for their judgment.

In another scenario, a wearable-based AI system analyzes patient data to flag potential health issues. Regulators require ongoing privacy protections and a clear plan for data sharing. The team writes a strict data-use policy, implements access controls, and commits to regular safety reviews. They also publish high-level summaries of performance and limitations for clinicians and patients, so everyone understands the tool's role and boundaries.

Liability, informed consent, and patient autonomy in AI-enabled care

Liability is the question of who is responsible when something goes wrong. In AI-enabled care, responsibility can be shared among clinicians, health systems, and technology providers. Clear agreements about roles help prevent finger-pointing in the moment of trouble. The central idea is that patients deserve clarity about who is making decisions and who is accountable for safety and outcomes.

Step 1: Clarify responsibilities among clinicians, institutions, and developers. Document who is responsible for patient decisions, for monitoring performance, and for updating the tools. When everyone knows their role, it's easier to manage risk and learn from mistakes.

Step 2: Communicate AI's role to patients and obtain informed consent where appropriate. Explain in plain language what the AI system does, what it does not do, and how clinicians will use its input. If a patient can reasonably be affected by AI guidance, offer a clear consent process and an opportunity to ask questions. The goal is transparency, not confusion.

Step 3: Ensure human oversight and the ability to override. AI tools should support clinicians, not replace them. Provide a straightforward way to review AI recommendations, adjust decisions, and rely on professional judgment when needed. The human-in-the-loop approach protects patient safety and preserves clinical responsibility.

Step 4: Keep transparent audit logs and explanations. When a decision is made, there should be accessible notes about why the AI suggested a certain action and how that suggestion was integrated with clinical judgment. This helps with accountability and learning from errors.

Step 5: Protect patient autonomy and offer opt-out options. Patients should have a voice in their care. If a patient prefers not to have AI assistance, offer alternatives that respect their choice. Autonomy means patients control over their own medical journey.

Step 6: Provide remediation for errors and ongoing training. When mistakes happen, investigate, learn, and update practices. Share findings with the care team and adjust workflows to prevent repeat issues. A culture of improvement reduces risk over time.

Two micro-cases to illustrate

In a hospital, a clinician uses an AI tool to help decide on a treatment plan. The clinician explains the AI input to the patient, discusses options, and confirms that the final decision rests with the clinician. The patient signs a consent form that mentions AI assistance. If a misstep occurs, the team reviews the case, learns from it, and strengthens both the tool and the process.

In a different setting, a patient receives an automated alert about a possible issue from a remote-monitoring AI. The alert triggers a clinician review, and the patient is informed about how the alert was generated and how their data was used. If the patient chooses to opt out of AI-driven monitoring, clinicians provide alternatives while continuing to monitor health through other means. The approach respects autonomy while maintaining safety nets.

Key Takeaway: Fairness, regulation, and patient rights are ongoing commitments; you build safer AI by planning for bias checks, proving safety and privacy to regulators, and keeping patients informed and in control.

Coming up next Subtittle: How to Get Started: Learning, Resources, and Roadmaps 1) Building multidisciplinary teams and fostering clinician–engineer collaboration, 2) Selecting tools, datasets, vendors, and open-source platforms wisely, 3) Practical roadmap for pilots, evaluation metrics, and long-term sustainability

Chapter 10

How to Get Started: Learning, Resources, and Roadmaps

By the end of this chapter, you will know how to start AI projects in healthcare by building a practical, cross-disciplinary team, choosing tools and data with care, and laying out a pilot plan that can grow into real, lasting practice.

Building multidisciplinary teams and fostering clinician–engineer collaboration

You will collaborate with people who bring different strengths. Clinicians understand patient care workflows and safety. Engineers understand data, models, and systems. When you work together with clear aims, communication, and respect for each other's expertise, you can move from ideas to usable tools that actually help patients.

Step 1: Define a shared purpose and outcomes

Begin with a simple, patient-centered goal that your team agrees on. Write down what success looks like in terms of care improvements, safety, or workflow, not just technical milestones. The why should be clear to everyone, from the chief clinician to the data engineer.

Rationale: A shared purpose keeps everyone focused during tough moments and helps you avoid projects that sound fancy but don't move patient care forward.

Step 2: Align roles and responsibilities

Assign roles that fit each person's strengths: clinical lead, data lead, product owner, quality and safety sponsor, and a trusted end-user representative. Create lightweight governance so decisions can be made without endless meetings.

Rationale: Clear ownership reduces confusion and speeds up progress. When people know who makes what call, you avoid bottlenecks.

Step 3: Create a common language and rituals

Agree on basic terms, data definitions, and decision criteria. Establish regular check-ins, concise progress updates, and a shared channel for questions. Use plain language that both clinicians and engineers can understand.

Rationale: A shared language lowers friction. Regular rituals build trust, so people speak up early when things aren't working.

Step 4: Start small to build trust

Pick a modest, well-defined problem you can finish in a short time. Use it as a learning loop to test workflows, governance, and the collaboration itself before tackling bigger goals.

Rationale: Small successes demonstrate value, reveal gaps, and teach the team how to work together smoothly.

Step 5: Build feedback and iteration into the cycle

Design your work to collect quick feedback from end users and use it to refine the tool. Track how changes affect care processes, not just model metrics.

Rationale: Real-world feedback protects patient safety and helps you build something that fits real clinical work.

Step 6: Invest in cross-training and shadowing

Offer brief learning sessions where clinicians see data science basics and engineers observe clinical workflows. Shadowing helps both sides anticipate challenges and improves collaboration.

Rationale: Shared literacy reduces misinterpretation and speeds joint problem-solving.

Step 7: Document decisions and learnings

Keep lightweight records of key decisions, trade-offs, and what you learned. Build a playbook you can reuse for future projects.

Rationale: Documentation creates repeatable patterns, so your team doesn't relearn the same lessons with every new project.

Two micro-cases to illustrate the approach

Case A: A hospital team pairs a nurse leader with a data engineer to design a simple alert that flags potential dehydration in high-risk patients using basic EHR notes and vitals. They agree on a clear goal, assign a clinical lead and a data lead, and meet weekly. After a few iterations based on nurse feedback, the alert integrates into the daily rounds workflow and shows modest time savings for care teams and improved early recognition.

Case B: A radiology resident teams up with a software engineer to prototype an auto-annotation helper for report drafting. They start with a tightly scoped task, test within a single department, and use weekly demos to gather clinician input. The prototype helps radiologists save minutes per report and provides a transparent explanation for any suggested annotation, building trust and setting up a path for broader use.

Tools, templates, and quick-start guidance

- Team charter template: roles, goals, decision rights, meeting cadence, and a simple escalation path.

- Communication norms: channel for quick questions, a weekly demo, and a plain-language glossary.

- Collaboration checklist: one-page reminder of how the clinician and engineer will share feedback, handle conflicts, and celebrate small wins.

Selecting tools, datasets, vendors, and open-source platforms wisely

Choosing the right tools and datasets is not about chasing the latest trend. It's about matching capabilities to your goals, ensuring safety and privacy, and preserving the ability to learn and adapt over time. Make decisions that you can explain clearly to clinicians, administrators, and patients.

Step 1: Align tools with your goals and workflows

Ask what problem you're solving, who will use the tool, and how it fits into existing routines. Favor tools that integrate smoothly with current systems and support the tasks clinicians perform daily.

Rationale: If a tool makes care work harder or disrupts patient flows, it won't gain adoption, no matter how impressive the model might seem.

Step 2: Check data compatibility, quality, and provenance

Assess where the data comes from, how clean it is, and whether it can be trusted for clinical use. Favor data with clear origin, documented quality checks, and well-understood limits.

Rationale: High-quality data underpins reliable results and safer care.

Step 3: Prioritize safety, privacy, and compliance

Select tools with clear safeguards for patient data, strong access controls, and transparent handling of identifiers. Ensure alignment with applicable rules and standards your institution follows.

Rationale: Protecting patient privacy isn't optional; it's a fundamental part of care that keeps trust intact.

Step 4: Evaluate support, reliability, and learnability

Consider how easy the tool is to learn, how often it's updated, and what kind of help is available from vendors or the community. Favor options with good documentation and active support networks.

Rationale: A tool that's hard to learn or rarely updated slows you down and increases risk of bad outcomes.

Step 5: Weigh open-source versus commercial options

Open-source tools offer transparency and flexibility but may require more in-house work. Commercial solutions can provide speed and support but may lock you in. Balance openness with practical needs and ensure you retain rights to data and outcomes.

Rationale: A balanced portfolio reduces risk, gives you options, and supports long-term sustainability.

Step 6: Plan for interoperability and future-proofing

Choose architectures and standards that encourage easy data sharing and system integration. Favor modular designs that let you swap components as needs evolve.

Rationale: Interoperable systems prevent data silos and make expansion easier over time.

Two micro-cases to illustrate the choice process

Case A: A hospital evaluates open-source NLP tools to process discharge summaries. They pick widely used, well-documented components with strong community support, test on a small set of notes, and plan phased integration into the EHR. The team values transparency, easier troubleshooting, and the ability to customize features over time.

Case B: A startup looks for a cloud-based AI platform. They require strong data governance, clear ownership of results, and robust auditing. After comparing vendors, they choose a platform that promises clear data handling policies, predictable pricing, and documented integration points with their existing systems. The decision supports rapid prototyping while keeping patient trust front and center.

Practical roadmaps, pilots, metrics, and sustainability

A practical roadmap helps you turn ideas into reliable practice. Start with a clear, bounded pilot, then grow as you learn what works.

Step 1: Clarify the problem and define success

Describe the clinical problem, the expected care improvement, and the tangible outcomes you want to see. Create simple success criteria that clinicians can recognize and validate.

Rationale: Clear targets prevent scope creep and help you measure real impact.

Step 2: Design the pilot with sensible scope

Limit the pilot to a single unit or workflow, use a concise timeline, and specify the data you'll collect. Ensure frontline staff can participate without excessive burden.

Rationale: A focused pilot reduces risk and makes it easier to demonstrate value.

Step 3: Gather baseline data and establish a control

Collect information about current performance before you change anything. If possible, compare to a similar area not using the new tool.

Rationale: Baseline data let you see what changed and why.

Step 4: Run iterative cycles with clinician feedback

Release the pilot in small, manageable updates. Use quick feedback loops with end users to refine the approach and fix problems early.

Rationale: Iteration keeps the project aligned with real clinical needs and safety requirements.

Step 5: Measure results with predefined metrics

Track outcomes that matter for patients and care teams. Use simple dashboards and regular reviews to keep everyone informed.

Rationale: Transparent metrics show whether the pilot is delivering the intended benefits.

Step 6: Plan scale and integration into routine care

If the pilot succeeds, map out how to scale across units, how to fund ongoing maintenance, and how to integrate with existing workflows and IT systems.

Rationale: Sustainability comes from thoughtful planning for people, processes, and technology.

Step 7: Build a governance and sustainability plan

Define roles for ongoing oversight, quality assurance, and continuous improvement. Include training, budgeting, and a long-term roadmap.

Rationale: A solid plan prevents backsliding once the initial excitement fades.

Exercises you can do now

- Exercise 1: Draft a team charter for a cross-disciplinary AI project. Time: 30 minutes. Outcome: a one-page document that clarifies roles, goals, and decision rights.

- Exercise 2: List five candidate tools or datasets and justify fit for your target workflow. Time: 45

minutes. Outcome: a short evaluation table you can share with your team.

- Exercise 3: Create a 90-day pilot plan with milestones and success criteria. Time: 60 minutes. Outcome: a practical plan you can present to leadership.

- Exercise 4: Design a simple metrics dashboard with three clinical metrics and a way to track them. Time: 25 minutes. Outcome: a ready-to-run dashboard sketch you can implement.

Templates and quick-start tools

- Team Charter Template: goals, roles, decision rights, meeting cadence, escalation path.

- Tool & Data Evaluation Checklist: alignment with goals, data quality, privacy controls, support, interoperability, licensing.

- Pilot Plan Skeleton: problem statement, scope, data needs, success metrics, rollout steps, risk notes.

- Metrics Dashboard Sketch: three metrics, data source, update frequency, and a review point.

Key Takeaway: The strongest AI efforts start with people who can work well together, the right tools chosen for real clinical needs, and a clear, bounded plan you can actually execute.

Transition: In the next chapter, you'll dig into healthcare data types and management—how electronic health records, images, wearables, and genomic data fit into learning systems, and how to protect privacy while enabling powerful insights. You'll build on the teamwork and tool-selection mindset here as you shape the data foundations for responsible AI-enabled care.

Dear Reader,

Thank you for exploring this series focused on failures and the power of comeback stories. If you find value in these stories and believe in the importance of embracing setbacks as part of growth, we appreciate your support. Please consider sharing a positive review on the platform where you accessed this series.

Your feedback helps spread the message, inspiring more young readers to see challenges as opportunities and to believe in their potential. We understand that mistakes happen, and we thank you for your understanding.

www.ingramcontent.com/pod-product-compliance
Lightning Source LLC
LaVergne TN
LVHW022208200926
848481LV00006B/1898
* 9 7 9 8 2 9 5 5 3 5 5 1 2 *